Vitamin Rich Vegetables

Roby Jose Ciju

CONTENTS

1 INTRODUCTION

All vegetables are part of plant kingdom. Plant kingdom is first divided into FOUR sub-communities: Thallophyta; Bryophyta; Pteridophyta; and Spermatophyta. All the vegetables are part of the sub-community Spermatophyta. Spermatophyta has two divisions: Gymnosperms and Angiosperms. All vegetable plants belong to the group Angiosperms. Group Angiosperms has two 'Classes': Moncotyledoneae and Dicotyledoneae. 'Class' are further divided into 'Family', 'Genus', 'Species', and 'Subspecies', 'Cultivar' or 'Variety'.

Botanical Classification of Vegetables

Botanical classification of vegetables based on two basic classes Monocotyledoneae and Dicotyledonaeae is given below:

Monocotyledoneae	Dicotyledonaeae
Family: Amaryllidaceae	Family: Aizoaceae
Family: Liliaceae	Family: Chenopodiaceae
Family: Araceae	Family: Compositae
Family: Dioscoreaceae	Family: Convolvulaceae
	Family: Cruciferae
	Family: Cucurbitaceae
	Family: Euphorbiaceae
	Family: Leguminosae
	Family: Malvaceae
	Family: Polygonaceae
	Family: Solanaceae
	Family: Umbelliferae

Classification of Vegetables Based on Plant Parts Used as Food

Leaves, shoots, stems, immature fruits, flower parts, and underground parts of the plants are generally consumed as vegetables. Based on plant parts used as food, there are FOUR major groups of vegetables: Leafy Vegetables; Fruit Vegetables; Flower Vegetables; and Root Vegetables.

Leafy Vegetables : Edible parts are leaves, shoots and/or stems

Brassica vegetables such as Cabbage, Chinese cabbage, and Kohlrabi, Spinach greens such as New Zealand Spinach and Malabar spinach, Vegetable greens such as Collard greens, Mustard greens, Coriander greens, Beet greens, and Mint herbs, Fenugreek Leaves, Drumstick leaves, Curry leaves, Amaranth leaves and Salad vegetables such as Kale, and Lettuce

Fruit Vegetables: Edible parts are immature fruits

Beans and Peas which includes Fava beans, Cluster beans, and French beans; Gourds and Melons comprising of vegetables such as Cucumber, Pumpkin, Wax gourd, Towel gourd, and Bottle gourd; Tomato, Eggplant/Brinjal, Okra/Lady's finger , Papaya, Jackfruit, Mango, Breadfruit, Plantains and Chilli Peppers

Flower Vegetables: Edible parts are flowers, flower clusters and associated parts

Major flower vegetables are Broccoli flower clusters, Sesbania flowers, Pumpkin flowers, Calabash gourd flowers and Cauliflower

Root Vegetables and Bulbous Vegetables: Edible parts are underground stems, bulbs, tubers and other associated parts

Carrot, Turnip, Radish, Potato, Cassava/Tapioca, Colocasia/Taro and Yam, Beets, Sweet potato, and Bulbous vegetables such as Onion, garlic, fennel bulb, shallots and Garlic

For writing this booklet, nutrient data available at USDA Nutrient Database of over 150 vegetables were analyzed. All the vegetables studied had absolutely NIL cholesterol and caffeine. In fact most of the vegetables may be regarded as cholesterol-free and caffeine-free foods.

A list of the vegetables analyzed for this study is given below.

Asparagus spears	Lettuce-green leaf	Bitter gourd pods
Agar seaweed	Romaine lettuce	Bitter gourd leafy tips
Amaranth	Iceberg crisphead lettuce	Towel gourd/dishcloth gourd
Arugula	Butterhead lettuce	Wax gourd/chinese preserving melon
Baby zucchini	Celery	Cowpeas leafy tips
Beet greens	Chives	Cowpeas pods
Brussels sprouts	Parsley	Green peas
Broccoli flowers	Globe artichoke	Yard long bean
Broccoli leaves	Jerusalem artichoke	Snap beans
Calabash gourd flowers	Rhubarb leafstalks	Fava beans/broad beans
Colocasia leaves	Peppermint leaves	Turnip greens
Chrysanthemum leaves	Spearmint leaves	Beets
Collard greens	Jalapeno peppers	Yam
Dock	Crimini mushrooms	Potatoes
Dandelion greens	Portabella mushrooms	Turnips
Drumstick pods	Shiitake mushrooms	Radishes

Drumstick leaves	Oyster mushrooms	Green cabbage
Endive	Enoki mushrooms	Red cabbage
Fireweed leaves	Maitake mushrooms	Savoy cabbage
Fenugreek leaves	Morel mushrooms	Cauliflower
Grape leaves	Chanterelle mushrooms	Carrots
Garden cress	Hungarian peppers	Baby carrots
Irishmoss seaweed	Banana peppers	Radicchio
Knolkhol	Serrano peppers	Green tomatoes
Kelp seaweed	Green chilli peppers	Orange tomatoes
Kale leaves	Red chilli peppers	Yellow tomatoes
Laver seaweed	Spring onions/scallions	Taro/colocasia tuber
Malabar spinach	Shallots	Cassava
Mustard spinach	Salsify/vegetable oyster	Okra/lady's finger
Mustard greens	Radicchio	Pumpkin
Napa cabbage	Poke/pokeberry shoots	Cucumber
New Zealand spinach	Parsnip	Sweet potato
Pak choi	Sweet onions	Plantains
Pumpkin flowers	Young green onion tops	Jackfruit
Pumpkin leaves	Onions	Breadfruit
Purslane	Nopales	Mangoes
Spirulina seaweed	Leeks	Papayas
Sesbania flowers	Lambs quarters	Jicama/yambean
English spinach	Ginger root	Rutabagas
Scotch kale	Garlic	Tomatillos
Swisschard	Fennel bulb	White sweet corn
Sweet pepper red	Epazote	Yellow sweet corn
Sweet pepper	Dill weed	Cassava

yellow		
Sweet pepper green	Cilantro/coriander greens	Okra/lady's finger
Sweet potato leaves	Chicory greens	Pumpkin
Winged bean leaves	Celtuce	Cucumber
Watercress	Celeriac	Sweet potato
Wakame seaweed	Cardoon	Spaghetti squash
White button mushrooms	Borage	Acorn squash
Lettuce-red leaf	Butterbur or fuki	Scallop squash
Hubbard squash	Indian squash/navajo	Butternut squash
Crookneck and straightneck squash		

2 VITAMINS

We need vitamins in small quantities for healthy living and staying fit. Vitamins are required to regulate body metabolism and tissue building. Requirement of vitamins increases with the increase in age. Insufficient amount of vitamins in the body results in vitamin deficiency diseases. There are fat-soluble and water-soluble vitamins.

Fat Soluble Vitamins

Vitamin A, D, E, and K (ADEK) are fat-soluble vitamins. That means, surplus consumption of these vitamins gets deposited in body fat and therefore daily consumption of these vitamins are not required.

Water Soluble Vitamins

Vitamin B and C are known water-soluble vitamins. Body cannot store water soluble vitamins such as vitamin B and Vitamin C and therefore any surplus amount is eliminated from body through urine. Daily consumption of these vitamins is essential to stay healthy and young. Water-soluble vitamins may get destroyed while cooking. Hence vegetables containing vitamin B and Vitamin C must be cooked by steaming or grilling rather than by boiling or deep frying.

3 VITAMIN A

Vitamin A is also known as Retinol. It is essential for eye health. It also strengthens body's natural immune system. Vitamin A is also essential for tissue building, and skin health. Vitamin A deficiency results in night blindness, and drying of skin and eyes. Among popular root vegetables, carrots and sweet potatoes are found to have large amounts of vitamin A. Among gourds and melons, winter squashes such as butternut squash and pumpkins are rich in vitamin A. Among popular leafy vegetables, kale and spinach are found to be excellent source of vitamin A.

Excellent Source of Vitamin A

A list of the vegetables that are rich source of vitamin A is given below:

Vegetable	IU/100 g
Grape Leaves	27521
Carrots	16706
Broccoli Leaves	16000
Sweet Potato	14187
Baby Carrots	13790
Lambs Quarters	11600
Turnip Greens	11587
Butternut Squash	10630
Dandelion Greens	10161
Kale Leaves	9990
Mustard Spinach	9900

English Spinach	9377
Romaine Lettuce	8710
Poke/Pokeberry Shoots	8700
Pumpkin	8513
Parsley	8424
Winged Bean Leaves	8090
Malabar Spinach	8000
Dill Weed	7718
Drumstick Leaves	7564
Lettuce-Red Leaf	7492
Lettuce-Green Leaf	7405
Garden Cress	6917
Cilantro/Coriander Greens	6748
Fenugreek Leaves	6450
Beet Greens	6326
Swisschard	6116
Chicory Greens	5717
Laver Seaweed	5202
Collard Greens	5019
Colocasia Leaves	4825
Pak Choi	4468
New Zealand Spinach	4400
Chives	4353
Peppermint Leaves	4248
Borage	4200
Spearmint Leaves	4054
Dock	4000
Young Green Onion Tops	4000

Moderate Source of Vitamin A

A list of the vegetables that are moderate source of vitamin A is given below:

Vegetable	IU/100 g
Sweetpotato Leaves	3778
Fireweed Leaves	3598
Celtuce	3500
Butterhead Lettuce	3312
Watercress	3191
Sweetpepper Red	3131
Scotch Kale	3100
Mustard Greens	3024
Broccoli Flowers	3000
Amaranth	2917
Arugula	2373
Endive	2167
Pumpkin Flowers	1947
Pumpkin Leaves	1942
Chrysanthemum Leaves	1870
Bittergourd Leafy Tips	1734
Leeks	1667
Orange Tomatoes	1496
Cowpeas Pods	1369
Hubbard Squash	1367
Purslane	1320
Green Chilli Peppers	1179
Plantains	1127
Red Cabbage	1116
Mangoes	1082
Jalapeno Peppers	1078
Savoy Cabbage	1000

Poor Source of Vitamin A

Among the studied vegetables, mushrooms and seaweeds were found to be poor sources of vitamin A. Popular vegetables such as Onions, Potatoes, Garlic, Ginger, Radishes, Turnips, Shallots, Artichokes and Cauliflowers were also poor source of vitamin A. The presence of vitamin A in vegetables such as Calabash Gourd Flowers, Cassava, Rutabagas, Sweet Onions, White Sweet Corn, Sesbania Flowers, Salsify/Vegetable Oyster, Parsnip, Celeriac, Cardoon, Wax Gourd/Chinese Preserving Melon, Yellow Tomatoes, Breadfruit, and Indian Squash/Navajo was negligible.

4 VITAMIN B COMPLEX

Vitamin B complex contains Vitamin B1 (thiamine), B2 (riboflavin), B3 (Niacin or Nicotinic acid), B5 (Pantothenic acid), B6 (Pyridoxine), B7 (biotin), B9 (Folate/Folic acid) and B12 (Cobalamin).

Vitamin B1

Vitamin B1 is also known as Thiamine. It is essential for proper functioning of muscular and nervous systems. It also facilitates fatty acid production in the body and is essential for energy production within the body. Its deficiency disorder is called Beriberi, major symptoms of which is improper functioning of muscular and nervous systems.

Vegetables Rich in Thiamine or Vitamin B1

Vegetable	Mg/100 g
Winged Bean Leaves	0.833
Cowpeas Leafy Tips	0.354
Green Peas	0.266
Drumstick Leaves	0.257
Enoki Mushrooms	0.225
Spirulina Seaweed	0.222
Colocasia Leaves	0.209
Jerusalem Artichoke	0.2
Garlic	0.2
Okra/Lady's Finger	0.2
White Sweetcorn	0.2

Okra/Lady's Finger	0.2
Dandelion Greens	0.19
Bittergourd Leafy Tips	0.181
Lambsquarters	0.16
Sweetpotato Leaves	0.156
Yellow Sweetcorn	0.155
Cowpeas Pods	0.15
Maitake Mushrooms	0.146
Asparagus Spears	0.143
Acorn Squash	0.14
Brussels Sprouts	0.139
Fava Beans/Broad Beans	0.133
Chrysanthemum Leaves	0.13
Oyster Mushrooms	0.125
Yam	0.112
Kale Leaves	0.11
Breadfruit	0.11
Yardlong Bean	0.107
Jackfruit	0.105

Poor Sources of Thiamine

Among the studied vegetables, following were found to be poor sources of thiamine:
Purslane, Onions, Orange Tomatoes, Arugula, Tomatillos, Baby
Zucchini, Pumpkin Flowers, Iceberg Crisphead Lettuce, Sweet
Onions, Yellow Tomatoes, Dock, Grape Leaves, Napa Cabbage,
New Zea Land Spinach, Pak Choi, Swisschard, Jalapeno Peppers,
Bitter Gourd Pods, Wax Gourd/Chinese Preserving Melon, Turnips,
Spaghetti Squash, Fireweed Leaves, Beets, Young Green Onion
Tops, Baby Carrots, Calabash Gourd Flowers, Sweet Pepper Yellow,
Epazote, Mangoes, Amaranth, Cucumber, Ginger Root, Papayas,
Celery, Rhubarb Leafstalks, Cardoon, Butterbur or Fuki,
Jicama/Yambean, Indian Squash/Navajo, Radicchio, Irishmoss
Seaweed, Shiitake Mushrooms, Chanterelle Mushrooms, Nopales,
Radishes, Fennel Bulb, and Agar Seaweed.

Vitamin B2 or Riboflavin

Vitamin B2 is also called Riboflavin. It is essential for eye health, skin health, hair health and energy metabolism. It is a powerful antioxidant vitamin. It also helps in the activation of Vitamin B6 and Vitamin B4. Major deficiency symptoms include swelling and redness of mouth, lips, tongue and skin. Another deficiency is anaemia due the decreased RBC (red blood cell) count.

Vegetables Rich in Riboflavin

Vegetable	Mg/100 g
Drumstick Leaves	0.66
Winged Bean Leaves	0.60
Crimini Mushrooms	0.49
Irishmoss Seaweed	0.47
Colocasia Leaves	0.46
Laver Seaweed	0.45
Lambsquarters	0.44
White Button Mushrooms	0.40
Bittergourd Leafy Tips	0.36
Grape Leaves	0.35
Oyster Mushrooms	0.35
Epazote	0.35
Sweetpotato Leaves	0.35
Spirulina Seaweed	0.34
Poke/Pokeberry Shoots	0.33
Dill Weed	0.30
Fava Beans/Broad Beans	0.29
Peppermint Leaves	0.27
Dandelion Greens	0.26
Garden Cress	0.26
Maitake Mushrooms	0.24
Wakame Seaweed	0.23
Beet Greens	0.22

Salsify/Vegetable Oyster	0.22
Shiitake Mushrooms	0.22
Chanterelle Mushrooms	0.22
Morel Mushrooms	0.21
Enoki Mushrooms	0.20

Moderate Source of Riboflavin

Vegetable	Mg/100 g
English Spinach	0.19
Spearmint Leaves	0.18
Cowpeas Leafy Tips	0.18
Cilantro/Coriander Greens	0.16
Amaranth	0.16
Malabar Spinach	0.16
Fenugreek Leaves	0.15
Kelp Seaweed	0.15
Borage	0.15
Chrysanthemum Leaves	0.14
Asparagus Spears	0.14
Cowpeas Pods	0.14
Fireweed Leaves	0.14
Green Peas	0.13
Collard Greens	0.13
Kale Leaves	0.13
New Zealand Spinach	0.13
Portabella Mushrooms	0.13
Pumpkin Leaves	0.13
Watercress	0.12
Broccoli Flowers & Broccoli Leaves	0.12
Chives	0.12

Poor Sources of Riboflavin

Among the popular vegetables, Onions and Shallots, Sweet peppers/Bell peppers, Winter squashes, Ginger, Tomatoes and Potatoes were found to be poor sources of Riboflavin.

Presence of riboflavin in vegetables such as Cucumber, Fennel Bulb, Yam, Rhubarb Leafstalks, Leeks, Cardoon, Turnips, Savoy Cabbage, Breadfruit, Scallop Squash, Jicama/Yambean, Radicchio, Papayas, Young Green Onion Tops, Iceberg Crisphead Lettuce, Taro/Colocasia Tuber, Agar Seaweed, Calabash Gourd Flowers, Knolkhol, and Butterbur Or Fuki was nil or negligible.

Vitamin B3 or Niacin

Vitamin B3 is also called Niacin or Nicotinic acid. It is essential for skin health, proper functioning of nerves, and digestion. It also reduces blood cholesterol level and therefore risk of heart attack. Deficiency disorder is called Pellagra. Deficiency symptoms include rashes on the skin, dementia and diarrhoea. The more severe case of the deficiency leads to death.

Vegetables Rich in Niacin

Vegetable	Mg/100 g
Enoki Mushrooms	7.03
Maitake Mushrooms	6.59
Oyster Mushrooms	4.96
Fireweed Leaves	4.67
Portabella Mushrooms	4.49
Chanterelle Mushrooms	4.09
Shiitake Mushrooms	3.89
Crimini Mushrooms	3.80
White Button Mushrooms	3.61
Winged Bean Leaves	3.47
Grape Leaves	2.36
Morel Mushrooms	2.25
Fava Beans/Broad Beans	2.25
Drumstick Leaves	2.22
Green Peas	2.09

Moderate Source of Niacin

Vegetable	Mg/100 g
Tomatillos	1.85
Yellow Sweetcorn	1.77
Peppermint Leaves	1.71
White Sweet Corn	1.70
Wakame Seaweed	1.60
Dill Weed	1.57
Serrano Peppers	1.54
Colocasia Leaves	1.51
Laver Seaweed	1.47
Parsley	1.31
Scotch Kale and Jerusalem Artichoke	1.30
Jalapeno Peppers	1.28
Red Chilli Peppers and Banana Peppers	1.24

Poor Sources of Niacin

Among the studied vegetables, following were found to be poor sources of Niacin: Rhubarb Leafstalks, Cardoon, Savoy Cabbage, Radicchio, Radishes, Green Cabbage, Watercress, Shallots, Butterbur or Fuki, Jicama/Yambean, Indian Squash/Navajo, Sweet Onions, Iceberg Crisphead Lettuce, Onions, Cucumber and Agar Seaweed.

Vitamin B6

Vitamin B6 is also known as Pyridoxine. It is essential for fat metabolism and protein metabolism. It also helps in the production of RBCs and neurotransmitters. Vitamin B6 facilitates proper functioning of estrogen and testosterone hormones in the body. Deficiency symptoms include depression, improper functioning of immune system and sores in mouth.

Vegetables Rich in Vitamin B-6/Pyridoxine

Vegetable	Mg/100 g
Garlic	1.24
Drumstick Leaves	1.20
Bittergourd Leafy Tips	0.80
Fireweed Leaves	0.63
Hungarian Peppers	0.52
Red Chilli Peppers and Serrano Peppers	0.51
Jalapeno Peppers	0.42
Grape Leaves	0.40
Banana Peppers	0.36
Shallots	0.35
Jackfruit	0.33
New Zealand Spinach, Plantains and Potatoes	0.30
Sweetpepper Red, Shiitake Mushrooms and Yams	0.29
Colocasia Tubers, Green Chilli Peppers and Salsify	0.28
Lambsquarters and Kale	0.27
Turnip Greens	0.26
Dandelion Greens	0.25

Poor Sources of Vitamin B-6

Among the studied vegetables, following were found to be poor sources of vitamin B-6: Celtuce, Fennel Bulb, Chanterelle Mushrooms, Bitter Gourd Pods, Towel Gourd, Iceberg Lettuce, Yambean, Calabash Gourd Flowers, Cucumber, Papayas, Wax Gourd, Spirulina Seaweed, Agar Seaweed, Rhubarb Leafstalks, Yardlong Bean, Endive, Kelp Seaweed, Wakame Seaweed, Fenugreek Leaves, Pumpkin Flowers, and Sesbania Flowers.

Vitamin B9 or Folate

It is also called Folic acid or Folate. It is essential for energy production from food. It helps in synthesis of nucleic acids and proper functioning of immune system and blood production by facilitating functioning of iron and increasing production of RBCs. It also helps in controlling amino acid metabolism.

Major deficiency symptoms include birth defects in new born babies, diarrhoea, hearing loss due to ageing, improper functioning of immune system, weakness, fatigue and headaches. Regular consumption of folic acid helps in slowing down progression of hearing loss with ageing; to prevent birth related defects in new born babies; for protection from cancer, heart diseases, depression and degeneration of body due to ageing; and to prevent memory loss and osteoporosis.

Vegetables Rich in Folate

All popular leafy vegetables such as spinach, parsley, kale, collard greens, chives and amaranth were found to be excellent source of folate. Popular seaweeds such as wakame, kelp, and irishmoss were also rich in folate content.

Vegetable	µg/100 g
Epazote	215
Wakame Seaweed	196
English Spinach and Turnip Greens	194
Irishmoss Seaweed	182
Kelp Seaweed	180
Chrysanthemum Leaves	177
Mustard Spinach	159
Parsley	152
Dill Weed	150
Fava Beans/Broad Beans	148
Laver Seaweed	146

Endive	142
Kale Leaves	141
Malabar Spinach	140
Romaine Lettuce	136
Collard Greens	129
Bittergourd Leafy Tips	128
Colocasia Leaves	126
Peppermint Leaves	114
Fireweed Leaves	112
Chicory Greens	110
Beets	109
Chives and Spearmint Leaves	105
Sesbania Flowers	102
Cowpeas Leafy Tips	101

Moderate Source of Folate

Vegetable	µg/100 g
Arugula	97
Agar Seaweed and Amaranth	85
Grape Leaves	83
Garden Cress and Savoy Cabbage	80
Napa Cabbage	79
Butterhead Lettuce	73
Bittergourd Pods	72
Broccoli Flowers and Leaves	71

Poor Sources of Folate

Among the studied vegetables, following were found to be poor sources of folate: Sweet Pepper Green, Butterbur Or Fuki, Spirulina Seaweed, Watercress, Green Tomatoes, Celeriac, Rhubarb Leafstalks, Towel Gourd/Dishcloth Gourd, Cucumber, Tomatillos, Cucumber, Calabash Gourd Flowers, Wax Gourd/Chinese Preserving Melon, Nopales, Garlic, Chanterelle Mushrooms, Sweet Potato Leaves, Fenugreek Leaves, Sweet Onions, Lettuce-Red Leaf, Shiitake Mushrooms, Morel Mushrooms, and Indian Squash/Navajo.

Vitamin B12

Vitamin B12 is also called Cobalamin. It helps in the synthesis of nucleic acids (DNA and RNA), RBCs and energy metabolism. Deficiency symptoms include loss of appetite, anaemia, constipation, and depression. It is sometimes used as a remedy for asthma, male infertility, heart disorders and cancer.

Vegetable Sources of Vitamin B 12

Among all the vegetables analyzed, only mushrooms are found to contain Vitamin B-12 in them. List of the mushrooms along with their Vitamin B 12 presence is given below:

Vegetable	µg/100 g
Crimini Mushrooms	0.1
Portabella Mushrooms	0.05
White Button Mushrooms	0.04

5 VITAMIN C

Vitamin C is also known as ascorbic acid. It is a powerful antioxidant vitamin. Vitamin C helps in absorption of iron and calcium. It increases body's natural immunity. Vitamin C deficiency results in a disease called scurvy. Major symptoms of scurvy are bleeding gum, joint pain, and hair loss.

Vegetables Rich in Vitamin C

Among popular vegetables, chilli peppers and bell peppers, broccoli and brussels sprouts, dark leafy greens such as kale and spinach and drumstick were found to be rich in vitamin C content.

Vegetable	Mg/100 g
Green Chilli Peppers	242.5
Sweet Pepper Yellow	183.5
Red Chilli Peppers	143.7
Drumstick Pods	141
Poke/Pokeberry Shoots	136
Parsley	133
Mustard Spinach and Scotch Kale	130
Sweetpepper Red	127.7
Kale Leaves	120
Jalapeno Peppers	118.6
Malabar Spinach	102
Broccoli Flowers and Leaves	93.2
Hungarian Peppers	92.9

Mushrooms and seaweeds were found to be a poor source of Vitamin C.

6 VITAMIN D

Vitamin D is essential for bone health. Its deficiency results in rickets which is weakening of bones in children and softening of bones in adults. The deficiency also results in osteoporosis and muscle weakening in adults.

Vegetables Rich in Vitamin D

Among the analyzed vegetables, only mushrooms are found to contain Vitamin D. In other words, mushrooms are the only source of Vitamin D in vegetable kingdom.

Vegetable	IU/100 g
Maitake Mushrooms	1123
Chanterelle Mushrooms	212
Morel Mushrooms	206
Oyster Mushrooms	29
Shiitake Mushrooms	18
Portabella Mushrooms	10
White Button Mushrooms	7
Enoki Mushrooms	5
Crimini Mushrooms	3

7 VITAMIN E

Vitamin E is essential for strengthening body's natural immune system and cardiovascular system. It is a powerful antioxidant vitamin and hence protects the body from heart diseases and cancer. Vitamin E deficiency results in weakening of muscular system and nervous system. Other deficiency symptoms include lack of coordination and balance.

Vegetables Rich in Vitamin E: Among popular vegetables, jalapenos, leafy vegetables such as cilantro, collard greens, spinach, swisschard and kale, winter squash and asparagus were found to be excellent source of vitamin E.

Vegetable	Mg/100 g
Jalapeno Peppers	3.58
Dandelion Greens	3.44
Turnip Greens	2.86
Cilantro/Coriander Greens	2.5
Taro/Colocasia Tuber	2.38
Collard Greens, Radicchio, Chicory Greens	2.26
English Spinach	2.03
Colocasia Leaves	2.02
Mustard Greens and Grape Leaves	2
Swisschard	1.89
Sweetpepper Red	1.58
Kale Leaves,	1.54
Beet Greens and Parsnip	1.5
Butternut Squash	1.44
New Zealand Spinach	1.42
Fava Beans/Broad Beans	1.16
Asparagus Spears	1.13
Pumpkin	1.06

Moderate Source of Vitamin E

Vegetable	Mg/100 g
Laver Seaweed, Watercress, Wakame Seaweed	1
Leeks	0.92
Mangoes	0.9
Brussels Sprouts	0.88
Agar Seaweed, Irishmoss, Kelp	0.87
Parsley	0.75
Garden Cress	0.7
Banana Peppers, Serrano Peppers, Chilli Peppers	0.69
Carrots	0.66
Fennel Bulb	0.58
Spring Onions/Scallions	0.55
Spirulina Seaweed and Cowpeas Pods	0.49
Knolkhol and Hungarian Peppers	0.48
Jicama/Yambean	0.46
Endive	0.44
Arugula	0.43
Snap Beans	0.41

Poor Sources of Vitamin E: Among the popular vegetables, Shallots and Onions, Beets, Turnips and Radishes, Cucumber, Mushrooms, Mints, Tomatoes and Potatoes, Amaranth, Baby Zucchini, Broccoli, Drumstick, Spinach, Kale and Sweet peppers were found to be poor sources of vitamin E.

Presence of vitamin E in vegetables such as Calabash Gourd Flowers, Chrysanthemum Leaves, Dock, Fireweed Leaves, Fenugreek Leaves, Pumpkin Flowers, Pumpkin Leaves, Purslane, Sesbania Flowers, Sweet Potato Leaves, Winged Bean Leaves, Nopales, Indian Squash/Navajo, Salsify/Vegetable Oyster, Poke/Pokeberry Shoots, Lambs Quarters, Epazote, Dill Weed, Celtuce, Cardoon, Borage, Butterbur Or Fuki, Bitter Gourd Pods, Bitter Gourd Leafy Tips, Wax Gourd/Chinese Preserving Melon, Cowpeas Leafy Tips, Yardlong Bean, Baby Carrots, and Acorn Squash was nil or negligible.

8 VITAMIN K

Vitamin K is essential for blood clotting, and for preventing heart diseases, cancer, and osteoporosis. Vitamin K deficiency results in bleeding gums and bleeding nose.

Vegetables Rich in Vitamin K

All popular dark green leafy vegetables, such as parsley, swisschard, kale, spinach, collard greens, and cilantro were rich in vitamin K. Vegetables like chives, lettuce and brussels sprouts were also found to be good source of vitamin K.

Vegetable	µg/100 g
Parsley	1640
Amaranth	1140
Swisschard	830
Dandelion Greens	778
Kale Leaves	705
Garden Cress	542
English Spinach	483
Collard Greens	437
Beet Greens	400
New Zealand Spinach	337
Cilantro/Coriander Greens	310
Sweetpotato Leaves	302

Moderate Source of Vitamin K

Vegetable	µg/100 g
Chicory Greens	298
Mustard Greens	258
Radicchio	255
Turnip Greens	251
Watercress	250
Endive	231
Chives	213
Spring Onions/Scallions	207
Brussels Sprouts	177
Young Green Onion Tops	156
Lettuce-Red Leaf	140
Lettuce-Green Leaf	126
Arugula, Colocasia Leaves, Grape Leaves	109
Romaine Lettuce	103
Butterhead Lettuce	102

Poor Sources of Vitamin K: Among the studied vegetables, sweet peppers, mushrooms and seaweeds, mints, squashes, yams and potatoes, sweet potatoes, tomatoes, onions and shallots, sweet corn, beets, radishes and turnips, ginger and garlic, drumsticks, spinach, kale, raw mangoes and papayas, and plantains were found to be poor sources of this vitamin. Vitamin K was absent in Jackfruit, Breadfruit, Knolkhol and Jerusalem artichoke also.

Other vegetables in which vitamin K was absent were Baby Carrots, Nopales, Cassava, Taro/Colocasia Tuber, Towel Gourd/Dishcloth Gourd, Jicama/Yambean, Rutabagas, Baby Zucchini, Broccoli Flowers, Broccoli Leaves, Calabash Gourd Flowers, Chrysanthemum Leaves, Dock, Fireweed Leaves, Fenugreek Leaves, Pumpkin Flowers, Pumpkin Leaves, Purslane, Winged Bean Leaves, Sesbania Flowers, Salsify/Vegetable Oyster, Poke/Pokeberry Shoots, Lambs Quarters, Epazote, Dill Weed, Celtuce, Cardoon, Borage, Butterbur Or Fuki, Bittergourd Pods, Bittergourd Leafy Tips, Wax Gourd/Chinese Preserving Melon, Cowpeas Leafy Tips, Yardlong Bean, Acorn Squash, and Indian Squash/Navajo.

9 CONCLUSION

Generally, people depend on food supplements for their necessary intake of vitamins and minerals. However, vitamin supplements or mineral supplements are not a substitute for a healthy diet. As we all know, a healthy diet is rich in fruits and vegetables. It is an established fact that natural intake of vitamins and minerals through a healthy diet increases human body's natural immunity and therefore prevents early incidences of many lifestyle diseases such as diabetes, heart diseases, stroke, cancer and obesity. Among vegetables, dark leafy greens such as Swiss chards, collard greens, kale, spinach, and mustard greens are considered to be nutrient-dense foods (i.e. foods rich in nutrients relative to the calories needed by a human body). Other nutrient dense foods among vegetables are broccoli and brussels sprouts, bell peppers (sweet peppers), sweet potatoes, cantaloupe, papayas, and mushrooms (crimini and shiitake).

ABOUT THE AUTHOR

Roby Jose Ciju is the author of '*The Art of Perfect Living*', an inspirational book based on scriptural wisdom. She is a professional horticulturist and an agribusiness consultant with a Masters Degree in Horticulture and a Post Graduate Diploma in Agri-Supply Chain Management. She has founded www.agrihortico.com, a website dedicated for publishing information on Food & Agriculture Topics. She has written more than 40 books on various Food & Agriculture topics till date and her best-selling books are, Mushroom Farming, Moringa, Curryleaf, Jalapeno Peppers, and Growing Ginger, Turmeric and Arrowroot. She may be contacted at roby@agrihortico.com. You may follow agrihortico at https://twitter.com/agrihortico1. Her official website is available at www.robyjoseciju.com.

Roby Jose Ciju

www.ingramcontent.com/pod-product-compliance
Lightning Source LLC
Chambersburg PA
CBHW010722110626
46523CB00046B/716